ALZHEIMER'S ATLAS

STRATEGIES IN ALZHEIMER'S DISEASE

MANAGEMENT

Dr. David O'Neill

Copyright

TABLE OF CONTENT

Introduction

Alzheimer's disease, a complex and devastating neurological disorder, has captured the attention of scientists, healthcare professionals, and society at large. In this introductory chapter, we embark on a journey to understand the essence of Alzheimer's, delving into its historical roots and pivotal discoveries that shaped our comprehension of this ailment.

Overview of Alzheimer's Disease

Alzheimer's disease, named after German psychiatrist and neurologist Alois Alzheimer, represents the most prevalent form of dementia globally. It is a progressive disorder that impairs memory, cognitive function, and eventually, the ability to carry out daily activities. The hallmark characteristics include the accumulation of beta-amyloid plaques and tau tangles in the brain, leading to neuronal damage and cognitive decline. To grasp the impact of Alzheimer's, it is crucial to recognize its prevalence and the staggering numbers of individuals affected. As populations age, the incidence of Alzheimer's rises, posing significant challenges to healthcare systems and societies. The emotional toll on families and caregivers cannot be overstated, making Alzheimer's a poignant and urgent global health concern.

Historical Context and Discoveries

The journey into understanding Alzheimer's begins in the early 20th century. In 1906, Dr. Alois Alzheimer first presented the case of Auguste Deter, a patient exhibiting profound memory loss and behavioral changes. Upon her death, Dr. Alzheimer examined her brain, revealing unusual pathology—neuritic plaques and neurofibrillary tangles. This seminal observation marked the identification of what we now recognize as Alzheimer's disease.

The subsequent decades witnessed incremental progress in comprehending Alzheimer's, with researchers gradually unraveling its intricacies. The advent of technology, particularly neuroimaging and genetic studies, brought new dimensions to our understanding. The discovery of the APOE ε4 gene's association with increased risk added a genetic component to the narrative, providing valuable insights into predisposition and susceptibility.

In the latter half of the 20th century, the development of biomarkers and advanced imaging techniques allowed researchers to visualize the progression of Alzheimer's pathology in living brains. This era also saw the formulation of diagnostic criteria, enabling earlier and more accurate identification of the disease. These milestones represented pivotal steps toward not only understanding Alzheimer's but also devising strategies for timely intervention.

The turn of the 21st century ushered in a surge of research focused on unraveling the molecular mechanisms underlying Alzheimer's pathology. Scientists explored the intricate interplay of various factors, including inflammation, synaptic dysfunction, and mitochondrial impairment. As the pieces of the puzzle came together, novel therapeutic targets emerged, offering hope for future treatments.

Collaboration across disciplines became increasingly crucial in the quest for a comprehensive understanding of Alzheimer's. Neuroscientists, geneticists, clinicians, and pharmaceutical researchers joined forces to decipher the complexities of this multifaceted disorder. Initiatives like the Alzheimer's Disease

Neuroimaging Initiative (ADNI) fostered large-scale data collection, paving the way for more robust research and clinical trials.

In recent years, breakthroughs in biomarker identification, coupled with advances in artificial intelligence, have accelerated the pace of Alzheimer's research. Large-scale genomics projects and global collaborations continue to shed light on the genetic underpinnings and regional variations in Alzheimer's prevalence.

As we embark on this exploration of Alzheimer's disease, it is essential to acknowledge the resilience of those affected, the dedication of researchers, and the collective determination to confront this formidable challenge. This chapter sets the stage for a comprehensive journey through the landscape of Alzheimer's, from its historical roots to the cutting-edge discoveries shaping our approach to diagnosis, treatment, and care.

Chapter One

Understanding Alzheimer's

disease

Understanding Alzheimer's goes beyond recognizing its clinical manifestations; it involves a nuanced exploration of the causes, risk factors, and the intricate interplay of genetic and environmental influences that contribute to the onset of this progressive neurological disorder. At its core, Alzheimer's is characterized by the aggregation of beta-amyloid plaques and tau tangles in the brain, resulting in neuronal damage and cognitive decline. Unraveling the complexities of these pathological hallmarks is essential to comprehend the disease's progression through different stages.

Causes and risk factors add layers to the narrative of Alzheimer's. While age remains the primary risk factor, genetic predispositions, particularly the APOE ε4 allele, contribute significantly to susceptibility. Environmental factors such as cardiovascular health, education, and lifestyle choices also play pivotal roles, highlighting the intricate web of elements influencing Alzheimer's development.

Genetic and environmental influences further underscore the heterogeneity of Alzheimer's presentations. Familial Alzheimer's disease, linked to specific genetic mutations, contrasts with the more common sporadic forms. Early-onset Alzheimer's, often rooted in genetic factors, diverges from the late-onset variety, where genetic predispositions interact with environmental elements over time.

Navigating the neurobiology of Alzheimer's adds depth to understanding its intricacies. A grasp of brain structure and function aids in deciphering the impact of pathological changes on cognitive processes. From synaptic dysfunction to neurotransmitter imbalances, each facet contributes to the overall deterioration observed in Alzheimer's patients.

As we embark on the journey of understanding Alzheimer's, this chapter serves as a foundation, fostering a comprehensive grasp of the disease beyond its surface-level symptoms. The intricate weave of genetic, environmental, and neurobiological elements invites us to explore Alzheimer's as a multifaceted challenge, laying the groundwork for the subsequent chapters on diagnosis, treatment, and caregiving.

Causes of Alzheimer's Disease

The causes of Alzheimer's disease are complex, involving a combination of genetic, environmental, and lifestyle factors. While the exact etiology remains elusive, scientific research has provided valuable insights into the mechanisms that contribute to the development of this neurodegenerative disorder.

Genetic Factors

APOE Gene:The apolipoprotein E (APOE) gene is a well-established genetic risk factor for Alzheimer's. Specifically, the APOE ε4 allele is associated with an increased risk of developing the disease. Individuals carrying one or two copies of this allele face a higher likelihood of Alzheimer's onset and often exhibit earlier symptoms.

Other Genetic Variants

Beyond APOE, ongoing genomic research continues to identify additional genetic variants linked to Alzheimer's susceptibility. These variations contribute to the complex genetic landscape, influencing the age of onset and severity of the disease.

Environmental Factors

❖ **Cardiovascular Health:** Conditions affecting cardiovascular health, such as hypertension, diabetes, and high cholesterol, have been implicated as potential contributors to Alzheimer's disease. The intricate relationship between vascular health and cognitive function underscores the importance of addressing cardiovascular risk factors in Alzheimer's prevention.

❖ **Educational and Cognitive Engagement:** Studies suggest a correlation between higher levels of education and cognitive engagement with a reduced risk of Alzheimer's. Intellectual stimulation throughout life may create a cognitive reserve, potentially delaying the onset of symptoms or mitigating their impact.

❖ **Traumatic Brain Injury (TBI):** A history of traumatic brain injury, especially repeated concussions, has been identified as a potential risk factor for Alzheimer's. The cumulative effects of TBI on the brain's structure and function may contribute to the development of neurodegenerative disorders later in life.

Risk Factors for Alzheimer's Disease

Understanding the risk factors associated with Alzheimer's provides a crucial framework for preventive measures and early intervention. While age is the most significant risk factor, various elements, ranging from genetics to lifestyle choices, contribute to an individual's susceptibility to this progressive neurological condition.

Age

- **Advancing Age:** Alzheimer's prevalence increases with age, making age the single most influential risk factor. While the disease can affect individuals in their 40s and 50s, the risk substantially rises after the age of 65. As life expectancy continues to increase, addressing Alzheimer's becomes an increasingly pressing concern.

Genetics

- **Family History:** A family history of Alzheimer's disease can elevate an individual's risk. While most cases are sporadic, a hereditary component exists, with certain genetic mutations increasing susceptibility. Individuals with first-degree relatives diagnosed with Alzheimer's may face a higher risk themselves.

- **APOE Gene:** The APOE ε4 allele, identified in the causes section, not only plays a role in the disease's development but is also a key genetic risk factor. The number of copies of this allele influences the degree of risk, with two copies amplifying the likelihood of Alzheimer's onset.

Lifestyle and Health Factors

- **Cardiovascular Health:** Conditions such as heart disease, high blood pressure, and diabetes are associated with an increased risk of Alzheimer's. Addressing and managing these cardiovascular risk factors may contribute to cognitive health and potentially reduce the risk of developing the disease.

- **Diet and Exercise:** Unhealthy dietary patterns and sedentary lifestyles have been linked to a higher risk of Alzheimer's. Conversely, adopting a balanced diet and engaging in regular physical activity may promote brain health and mitigate some risk factors.

- **Social and Cognitive Engagement:** Limited social interaction and cognitive stimulation are risk factors for Alzheimer's. Maintaining an active and socially engaged lifestyle, as well as participating in intellectually stimulating activities, may contribute to cognitive resilience.

As we explore the causes and risk factors associated with Alzheimer's disease, it becomes evident that this multifaceted condition demands a comprehensive understanding of genetic, environmental, and lifestyle influences. This knowledge not only enhances our comprehension of the disease but also lays the groundwork for targeted prevention and intervention strategies.

Chapter Two

Clinical Manifestations of

Alzheimer's Disease

Clinical manifestations of Alzheimer's disease unfold in a progressive manner, encompassing a spectrum of cognitive and functional impairments. Early signs often involve subtle memory lapses, such as forgetting recent conversations or misplacing items. As the disease advances, individuals may struggle with familiar tasks, experience language difficulties, and face challenges in problem-solving.

A defining characteristic of Alzheimer's is the progression through distinct stages. In the mild cognitive impairment (MCI) stage, cognitive decline is noticeable but doesn't yet severely impact daily life. Moderate Alzheimer's brings more pronounced symptoms, including difficulty

with basic activities and heightened confusion. In the severe stage, individuals often lose the ability to communicate, recognize loved ones, and independently carry out routine tasks.
Behavioral changes accompany cognitive decline, with mood swings, agitation, and withdrawal becoming common. The gradual erosion of cognitive functions profoundly affects not only individuals with Alzheimer's but also places a significant emotional and practical burden on their caregivers. Understanding the nuanced clinical manifestations is pivotal for timely diagnosis, appropriate care planning, and the development of interventions to enhance the quality of life for those affected by this challenging neurological condition.

Early signs and symptoms of Alzheimer's disease

Early signs and symptoms of Alzheimer's disease are subtle but represent the initial indicators of cognitive decline. Recognizing these early clues is crucial for timely diagnosis and intervention, allowing for better management and support for individuals affected by the disease.

➤ **Memory Loss:** One of the hallmark early signs is memory loss, particularly for recently learned information. Individuals may struggle to recall names, appointments, or recent conversations. Forgetfulness becomes more noticeable, and they may repeatedly ask for the same information.

➤ **Difficulty with Familiar Tasks:** Early on, individuals with Alzheimer's may find it challenging to perform tasks that were once routine. This can include everyday activities like cooking, managing finances, or using household appliances. The struggle with familiar tasks becomes apparent to those close to them.

➤ **Changes in Planning and Problem-Solving:** Individuals may experience difficulties in planning and problem-solving. Simple tasks, such as following a recipe or organizing a schedule, become more challenging. These cognitive changes may interfere with their ability to handle complex situations effectively.

➢ **Confusion with Time and Place:** Losing track of time, forgetting dates, and becoming disoriented about the current location are common early signs. Individuals may find it challenging to comprehend the passage of time or may forget how they arrived at a particular place.

➢ **Language Challenges:** Early language difficulties manifest as struggles to find the right words, repeat phrases, or join and maintain a coherent conversation. Individuals may also have trouble understanding spatial relationships, leading to challenges in reading or judging distances.

➢ **Misplacing Items:** Misplacing belongings and being unable to retrace steps to find them is a common early symptom. This goes beyond occasional absent-mindedness, and individuals may put things in unusual places, forget where they put them, and struggle to retrace their steps.

➢ **Changes in Mood and Personality:** Early signs of Alzheimer's can include shifts in mood and personality. Individuals may become more irritable, anxious, or withdrawn. These changes are often noticeable to family and friends who are familiar with their usual demeanor. Recognizing these early signs empowers individuals and their loved ones to seek medical evaluation promptly. While these symptoms alone do not definitively diagnose Alzheimer's, they warrant attention and further assessment by healthcare professionals. Early intervention can lead to more effective management strategies and support, improving the overall quality of life for those affected by Alzheimer's disease.

Progression through different stages of Alzheimer's Disease

Alzheimer's disease progresses through distinct stages, each marked by specific cognitive and functional changes. Understanding these stages is crucial for caregivers, healthcare professionals, and individuals affected, as it shapes care strategies and informs expectations throughout the course of the disease.

1. **Preclinical Stage:** In the preclinical stage, individuals show no outward signs of

cognitive decline. However, subtle changes are occurring at the cellular and molecular levels in the brain. Advances in biomarker research aim to identify these changes, allowing for early intervention strategies.

2. **Mild Cognitive Impairment (MCI):** The onset of MCI is characterized by noticeable cognitive decline that is beyond what is expected for a person's age but not severe enough to impact daily life. Memory lapses and difficulties with complex tasks become evident. Not everyone with MCI progresses to Alzheimer's, but it is considered a risk factor.

3. **Early-Stage Alzheimer's:** Early-stage Alzheimer's is marked by mild cognitive decline that begins to affect daily activities. Memory deficits become more apparent, and individuals may have trouble recalling names, organizing thoughts, or completing familiar tasks. Despite these challenges, individuals in this stage can often function independently with some support.

4. **Moderate-Stage Alzheimer's:** As the disease progresses to the moderate stage, cognitive decline becomes more

pronounced. Individuals may struggle with basic activities such as dressing, bathing, and managing personal hygiene. Memory loss intensifies, and they may exhibit confusion about time, place, and people. Behavioral changes, including agitation and aggression, can emerge.

5. **Severe-Stage Alzheimer's:** In the severe stage, individuals experience a profound loss of cognitive and physical function. Communication becomes severely impaired, with a decline in language skills and the ability to recognize loved ones. Motor skills deteriorate, and individuals may become bedridden. Full-time assistance is required for basic daily activities.

Navigating these stages involves adapting care approaches to address evolving needs. Early-stage interventions may focus on maintaining independence and cognitive stimulation. In the moderate stage, personalized care plans should consider safety concerns and provide structured routines. In the severe stage, a focus on comfort, quality of life, and support for both the individual and their caregivers becomes paramount.

Progression through these stages is highly individualized, and the duration of each stage can vary. It's important for caregivers to engage in open communication with healthcare professionals to tailor care strategies to the unique needs and challenges faced by individuals with Alzheimer's disease. Additionally, ongoing research seeks to identify targeted interventions that may slow or modify the progression of the disease, offering hope for improved outcomes in the future.

Chapter Three

Diagnosis and Assessment of

Alzheimer's Disease

Diagnosing Alzheimer's disease involves a comprehensive assessment that considers medical history, cognitive tests, and imaging studies. Early diagnosis is crucial for effective management and support. Healthcare professionals often begin with a thorough evaluation, ruling out other potential causes for cognitive decline. Cognitive assessments, including memory and problem-solving tests, help determine the extent of impairment. Biomarker tests, such as cerebrospinal fluid analysis and brain imaging (MRI or PET scans), aid in detecting Alzheimer's-specific changes in the brain. Collaborative efforts between healthcare providers, neurologists, and neuropsychologists ensure a holistic approach to diagnosis. While there is no cure for Alzheimer's, an accurate and timely diagnosis empowers individuals and their families to plan for the future, access appropriate resources, and explore available treatment options to enhance quality of life.

Diagnostic tools and procedures for Alzheimer's Disease

Diagnosing Alzheimer's disease involves a multi-faceted approach, combining clinical evaluations, cognitive assessments, and advanced diagnostic tools. Timely and accurate diagnosis is essential for effective management, support, and future planning. Here, we explore the primary diagnostic tools and procedures used in identifying Alzheimer's disease.

> ➤ **Clinical Assessment:** A thorough clinical evaluation is the initial step in diagnosing Alzheimer's. Healthcare professionals gather a detailed medical history, including family history of cognitive disorders. They assess cognitive function, behavioral changes, and daily functioning.

Observations from family members or caregivers play a crucial role in understanding the individual's cognitive decline.

➢ **Cognitive Testing:** Specialized cognitive tests are employed to assess memory, attention, language, and problem-solving skills. The Mini-Mental State Examination (MMSE) and Montreal Cognitive Assessment (MoCA) are commonly used tools. These tests provide a quantitative measure of cognitive abilities and help determine the severity of impairment.

➢ **Biomarker Testing:** Biomarkers are biological indicators that can reveal underlying pathological changes associated with Alzheimer's disease. Cerebrospinal fluid analysis involves assessing levels of proteins like beta-amyloid and tau, which are indicative of Alzheimer's pathology. Blood tests are also being explored for potential biomarkers, offering a less invasive option.

➢ **Neuroimaging:** Advanced imaging techniques provide detailed insights into brain structure and function. Magnetic

Resonance Imaging (MRI) scans detect changes in brain structure, while Positron Emission Tomography (PET) scans, using tracers like florbetapir or flutemetamol, visualize beta-amyloid plaques. Functional MRI (fMRI) assesses brain activity, aiding in understanding the impact of Alzheimer's on neural networks.

➢ **Genetic Testing:** Genetic testing, particularly for the APOE gene, helps identify genetic predispositions linked to Alzheimer's risk. While having the APOE ε4 allele increases susceptibility, it doesn't guarantee the development of the disease. Genetic testing aids in assessing the overall risk profile.

➢ **Neuropsychological Evaluation:** Neuropsychological assessments provide a comprehensive evaluation of cognitive functions, including memory, attention, language, and executive function. These in-depth evaluations help in identifying specific cognitive deficits and patterns characteristic of Alzheimer's disease.

➢ **Functional Assessment:** Evaluating an individual's ability to perform daily activities is crucial. Functional assessments assess the impact of cognitive decline on tasks such as dressing, bathing, and meal preparation. This provides valuable information for care planning and understanding the individual's level of independence.

➢ **Collaborative Approach:** Diagnosing Alzheimer's often involves a collaborative effort among healthcare professionals. Neurologists, neuropsychologists, geriatricians, and other specialists contribute their expertise to ensure a comprehensive assessment. Interdisciplinary collaboration enhances diagnostic accuracy and aids in tailoring interventions.

While there is no definitive single test for Alzheimer's, the combination of these diagnostic tools enhances accuracy. It's important to note that diagnosis is not a one-size-fits-all process, and individual variations in presentation and progression are considered. Early and accurate diagnosis empowers individuals and their families to make informed decisions, access appropriate support services, and participate in research studies aimed at advancing our understanding and treatment of Alzheimer's disease.

Importance of early detection in

Alzheimer's Disease

The importance of early detection in Alzheimer's disease cannot be overstated, as it significantly influences the course of the disease and the overall well-being of individuals and their families.

✓ **Early Intervention and Treatment:** Early detection allows for prompt intervention and access to available treatments that may help manage symptoms and slow the progression of Alzheimer's. While there is no cure, medications such as cholinesterase inhibitors and memantine are more effective when initiated in the early stages.

✓ **Care Planning:** Early diagnosis enables individuals and their families to engage in comprehensive care planning. This involves addressing safety concerns, legal and financial matters, and making decisions about long-term care. Planning at the early stages provides a clearer roadmap for navigating the challenges associated with Alzheimer's.

✓ **Quality of Life:** Early detection positively impacts the quality of life for individuals with Alzheimer's. It allows them to actively participate in decisions about their care, express preferences, and engage in meaningful activities while they still have a higher level of cognitive function.

✓ **Emotional and Psychological Support:** An early diagnosis opens the door to emotional and psychological support for both the individual and their caregivers. Understanding the nature of the disease early on facilitates coping strategies, reduces uncertainty, and fosters a supportive environment that can mitigate the emotional impact of the diagnosis.

✓ **Participation in Clinical Trials:** Early detection enables individuals to consider participating in clinical trials and research studies exploring potential treatments and interventions. Active involvement in research contributes to the advancement of our understanding of Alzheimer's and may offer access to cutting-edge therapies.

✓ **Reduced Caregiver Burden:** Early diagnosis provides an opportunity for caregivers to receive education, training, and support services tailored to the specific needs of individuals with Alzheimer's. This proactive approach helps reduce caregiver burden and enhances their ability to provide effective and compassionate care.

✓ **Delayed Institutionalization:** With early detection and proper management, individuals with Alzheimer's may experience a delay in the need for institutional care. The ability to remain in familiar surroundings for a more extended period contributes to a higher quality of life and greater independence.

In essence, early detection empowers individuals and their support networks to face the challenges of Alzheimer's with knowledge, preparedness, and access to available resources. It transforms the trajectory of the disease from uncertainty and crisis management to proactive planning, ensuring that individuals with Alzheimer's can live fuller and more engaged lives for as long as possible.

Chapter Four

Types of Alzheimer's Disease

Alzheimer's disease manifests in various forms, with two primary types; sporadic (late-onset) and familial (early-onset). Sporadic Alzheimer's, accounting for the majority of cases, typically occurs after the age of 65 and lacks a clear genetic link. Familial Alzheimer's, on the other hand, is rare and hereditary, with onset often before 65. Mutations in specific genes like APP, PSEN1, and PSEN2 are associated with familial cases. Understanding these types helps unravel the diverse genetic and environmental factors contributing to the onset and progression of Alzheimer's disease.

Familial Alzheimer's disease

Familial Alzheimer's disease (FAD) represents a less common but more aggressive form of Alzheimer's, distinguished by a strong hereditary component. This variant typically affects individuals in their 30s, 40s, or 50s, well before the typical onset age for sporadic Alzheimer's.

Genetic Basis

FAD is primarily linked to mutations in three genes: Amyloid Precursor Protein (APP), Presenilin 1 (PSEN1), and Presenilin 2 (PSEN2). Mutations in these genes disrupt the normal processing of amyloid precursor protein, leading to the accumulation of beta-amyloid plaques—a hallmark of Alzheimer's pathology.

Inheritance Patterns

FAD follows an autosomal dominant inheritance pattern, meaning that an individual with a mutated gene has a 50% chance of passing it on to their offspring. If inherited, the mutation almost guarantees the development of Alzheimer's, often with a relatively predictable age of onset.

Symptoms and Progression

Familial Alzheimer's often progresses more rapidly than the sporadic form. Cognitive decline, memory loss, and behavioral changes manifest at an earlier age, impacting individuals in the prime of their lives. The symptoms mirror those of sporadic Alzheimer's but occur at an accelerated pace.

Impact on Families

FAD has profound implications for affected families. Witnessing the cognitive decline of a parent or sibling at a relatively young age poses unique challenges emotionally, financially, and socially. Family members may opt for genetic testing to determine their risk, which can bring about complex decisions and emotions.

Research and Treatment

Familial Alzheimer's has become a focal point in Alzheimer's research due to its clear genetic link. Studying families with FAD has led to crucial insights into the underlying mechanisms of Alzheimer's disease. While there is no cure, ongoing research aims to develop targeted treatments to delay or prevent the onset of symptoms.

Understanding familial Alzheimer's provides a window into the intricate interplay of genetics in this complex neurological disorder. Research advances in FAD not only contribute to understanding early-onset Alzheimer's but also hold promise for insights into the more common sporadic form, offering hope for innovative treatments and interventions.

Early-onset vs. late-onset Alzheimer's Disease

Alzheimer's disease can be broadly classified into two main types based on the age of onset: early-onset Alzheimer's disease (EOAD) and late-onset Alzheimer's disease (LOAD). While both share common pathological features, they exhibit distinctions in terms of age, genetic factors, and clinical manifestations.

Early-Onset Alzheimer's Disease (EOAD)

Age of Onset
EOAD refers to cases where symptoms manifest before the age of 65. Individuals with EOAD often

experience cognitive decline during their 40s or 50s, impacting their professional and personal lives during a more active phase of adulthood.

Genetic Factors

EOAD has a stronger genetic component compared to LOAD. Mutations in specific genes are associated with familial Alzheimer's disease (FAD), a rare but hereditary form. The three main genes linked to FAD are Amyloid Precursor Protein (APP), Presenilin 1 (PSEN1), and Presenilin 2 (PSEN2).

Progression

EOAD tends to progress more rapidly than LOAD. The accelerated decline in cognitive function can be especially challenging for individuals, their families, and caregivers. Early symptoms often include memory loss, language difficulties, and impaired spatial skills.

Impact on Families

The impact of EOAD on families is profound, as it disrupts lives during a phase when individuals are typically active in their careers and raising families. Witnessing a loved one experience cognitive decline at a younger age adds unique emotional and practical challenges to caregiving.

Late-Onset Alzheimer's Disease (LOAD)

Age of Onset

LOAD, the more common form, occurs when symptoms develop after the age of 65. It is often associated with aging, and the risk increases significantly with each advancing decade. The majority of Alzheimer's cases fall into the LOAD category.

Genetic Factors

While genetic factors play a role in LOAD, they are not as deterministic as in EOAD. The APOE ε4 allele is a significant genetic risk factor for LOAD, but its presence doesn't guarantee the development of the disease. LOAD is considered a complex interplay between genetic, environmental, and lifestyle factors.

Progression

LOAD typically progresses more gradually than EOAD. Individuals may experience mild cognitive impairment before advancing to more severe stages. The slower progression allows for a more extended period of functional independence, but it presents challenges for early diagnosis.

Impact on Families

The impact of LOAD is widespread, affecting families as individuals age. While the disease may unfold more gradually, it poses long-term challenges for both individuals and their caregivers. Coping with the evolving cognitive decline and providing adequate support becomes a central focus for families.

Shared characteristics

Both early-onset and late-onset Alzheimer's share fundamental characteristics, including the accumulation of beta-amyloid plaques and tau tangles in the brain, leading to synaptic dysfunction and cognitive decline. The ultimate impact on memory, language, and daily functioning is consistent across both forms of the disease.

Understanding the distinctions between early-onset and late-onset Alzheimer's is crucial for accurate diagnosis, prognosis, and treatment planning.

Chapter Five

Neurobiology of Alzheimer's disease

Brain structures involved in Alzheimer's disease
Alzheimer's disease profoundly impacts the structure and function of the brain, causing widespread changes that underlie the cognitive decline characteristic of the condition.

1. **Hippocampus:** The hippocampus, a key region for memory formation and consolidation, is particularly vulnerable in Alzheimer's disease. This small, seahorse-shaped structure in the temporal lobe experiences early and severe atrophy, contributing to memory deficits observed in individuals with the condition.

2. **Cortex:** The cortex, comprising the outer layer of the brain, is responsible for higher cognitive functions, including reasoning, language, and perception. In Alzheimer's, cortical regions, especially the frontal and temporal lobes, undergo progressive degeneration, leading to impairments in executive function, language, and recognition.

3. **Amygdala:** The amygdala, critical for emotional processing and memory, is affected in Alzheimer's. Changes in the amygdala contribute to alterations in emotional regulation and may manifest as mood disturbances, such as anxiety and depression.

4. **Synapses and Neural Networks:** Synapses, the connections between neurons, are fundamental for communication within the brain. In Alzheimer's, the accumulation of beta-amyloid plaques and tau tangles disrupts synaptic function. This synaptic dysfunction impairs neural communication, leading to cognitive decline.

5. **Basal Forebrain:** The basal forebrain contains crucial structures, including the

nucleus basalis of Meynert, which produces acetylcholine, a neurotransmitter vital for memory and learning. In Alzheimer's, degeneration of the basal forebrain contributes to a significant reduction in acetylcholine levels, impacting cognitive functions.

6. **Default Mode Network (DMN):** The DMN, involved in self-referential thinking and memory consolidation, is altered in Alzheimer's disease. Disruptions in the DMN contribute to the characteristic decline in episodic memory and self-awareness observed in affected individuals.

Understanding these structural and functional changes provides insights into the diverse cognitive deficits seen in Alzheimer's disease.

Pathology of Alzheimer's disease

The pathology of Alzheimer's disease is characterized by distinct changes in the brain's structure and function, resulting in the progressive deterioration of cognitive abilities. Two primary hallmarks define the pathology: the accumulation of beta-amyloid plaques and the formation of tau protein tangles.

1. **Beta-Amyloid Plaques:** In Alzheimer's, beta-amyloid, a normal protein in the brain, undergoes abnormal processing. This leads to the formation of insoluble plaques that accumulate between nerve cells. These plaques consist of clusters of beta-amyloid peptides and trigger inflammatory responses, disrupting the communication between neurons and contributing to neuronal damage.

2. **Tau Protein Tangles:** Tau proteins play a crucial role in stabilizing microtubules within neurons, aiding in the transport of nutrients and cellular components. In Alzheimer's, tau proteins undergo abnormal modifications, causing them to aggregate into neurofibrillary tangles. These tangles disrupt the structural integrity of neurons, impair cellular function, and contribute to the progressive loss of cognitive abilities.

3. **Neuronal Damage and Cell Death:** The accumulation of beta-amyloid plaques and tau protein tangles leads to widespread neuronal damage and eventual cell death.

This degeneration is particularly prominent in brain regions associated with memory and cognitive functions, such as the hippocampus and cortex.

4. **Synaptic Dysfunction:** Synaptic dysfunction is a central feature of Alzheimer's pathology. As beta-amyloid plaques and tau tangles accumulate, communication between neurons at synapses is disrupted. This synaptic failure contributes significantly to the cognitive deficits observed in individuals with Alzheimer's disease.

5. **Inflammatory Responses:** The presence of beta-amyloid plaques triggers inflammatory responses from the brain's immune cells. While inflammation is initially a protective response, chronic activation can exacerbate neuronal damage and contribute to the neurodegenerative process in Alzheimer's.

Understanding the pathology of Alzheimer's is crucial for developing targeted interventions and therapies. Researchers explore various strategies, from reducing beta-amyloid accumulation to preventing tau tangle formation, with the goal of slowing or halting the progression of this devastating neurological disorder.

Chapter six

Treatment Approaches for

Alzheimer's disease

Treatment approaches for Alzheimer's disease aim to manage symptoms, slow cognitive decline, and enhance quality of life. Medications such as cholinesterase inhibitors (donepezil, rivastigmine, galantamine) and memantine are prescribed to improve neurotransmitter function and regulate glutamate levels, temporarily alleviating cognitive symptoms. However, these drugs do not halt disease progression. Non-pharmacological interventions include cognitive stimulation programs, physical exercise, and social engagement, which may provide cognitive benefits and enhance overall well-being.

Medications their effects on Alzheimer's disease

Medications play a crucial role in managing Alzheimer's disease, primarily aiming to alleviate symptoms, enhance cognitive function, and improve the overall quality of life for individuals affected. Two main classes of medications are commonly prescribed:

1. **Cholinesterase Inhibitors:** Medications like donepezil (Aricept), rivastigmine (Exelon), and galantamine (Razadyne) fall into this category. They work by increasing acetylcholine levels in the brain, a neurotransmitter crucial for memory and learning. While these drugs do not alter the course of the disease, they can temporarily improve cognitive symptoms and enhance daily functioning.

2. **Memantine:** Memantine (Namenda) is an N-methyl-D-aspartate (NMDA) receptor

antagonist. It regulates glutamate activity, preventing excessive stimulation that can lead to neuronal damage. Memantine is often prescribed in moderate to severe stages of Alzheimer's to help manage cognitive symptoms and maintain functional abilities.

While these medications provide symptomatic relief, it's important to note that they do not cure Alzheimer's or halt disease progression. The effects vary among individuals, and the response to medication can be influenced by factors such as overall health, the stage of the disease, and individual differences in drug metabolism.

Challenges and Considerations

Medications may have side effects, including gastrointestinal issues or changes in sleep patterns. Additionally, individual responses can differ, and not everyone experiences significant benefits. Balancing the potential benefits with side effects requires ongoing monitoring and adjustments by healthcare professionals.

Future Perspectives

Ongoing research explores new drug targets and disease-modifying treatments. Antibody-based therapies targeting beta-amyloid and tau, as well as anti-inflammatory drugs, are subjects of investigation. These potential treatments aim to address the underlying pathology of Alzheimer's, offering hope for more effective interventions in the future.

Non-pharmacological interventions in Alzheimer's Disease

Non-pharmacological interventions are integral components of the comprehensive approach to managing Alzheimer's disease, focusing on enhancing cognitive function, improving quality of life, and providing support for individuals and their caregivers.

- **Cognitive Stimulation:** Engaging in cognitive activities can stimulate neural networks and promote cognitive function. Activities such as puzzles, games, and reminiscence therapy encourage mental engagement, potentially slowing cognitive decline and fostering a sense of accomplishment.

- **Physical Exercise:** Regular physical activity has been linked to cognitive benefits. Exercise promotes blood flow to the brain, supports neuroplasticity, and contributes to overall well-being. Tailored exercise programs, including activities like walking, stretching, and strength training, are beneficial for individuals with Alzheimer's.

- **Social Engagement:** Maintaining social connections is crucial for emotional well-being. Social engagement reduces feelings of isolation and provides opportunities for communication and interaction. Group activities, community programs, and support groups offer valuable social experiences for individuals with Alzheimer's.

- **Music and Art Therapy:** Music and art therapies tap into creative expression and emotional memory. Listening to music or participating in art activities can evoke positive emotions, stimulate communication, and provide avenues for self-expression even as cognitive abilities decline.

- **Sensory Stimulation:** Activities that engage the senses, such as aromatherapy, tactile stimulation, or exposure to nature, can be calming and enjoyable for individuals with

Alzheimer's. Sensory experiences enhance overall well-being and contribute to a more positive and relaxed environment.

- **Caregiver Support and Education:** Providing support and education for caregivers is crucial. Caregiver training programs offer practical strategies for managing challenging behaviors, improving communication, and ensuring the safety and well-being of both individuals with Alzheimer's and their caregivers.

- **Environmental Modifications:** Creating a supportive environment involves making adjustments to accommodate the needs of individuals with Alzheimer's. This may include reducing clutter, ensuring safety measures, and maintaining a consistent daily routine to enhance familiarity and reduce anxiety.

Non-pharmacological interventions not only contribute to improving cognitive function but also address the emotional and psychological aspects of Alzheimer's for both individuals and their caregivers.

Chapter seven

Caregiving Challenges

Caregiving for individuals with Alzheimer's presents numerous challenges. Progressive cognitive decline requires caregivers to adapt continuously, managing changing needs and behaviors. Emotional stress, exhaustion, and social isolation are common among caregivers. Communication difficulties, mood swings, and the need for constant supervision pose additional challenges. Balancing care responsibilities with personal well-being is demanding, emphasizing the importance of caregiver support, education, and respite care to alleviate the significant challenges associated with caring for those with Alzheimer's disease.

Emotional impact on caregivers

The emotional impact on caregivers of individuals with Alzheimer's disease is profound, encompassing a range of feelings that evolve as the disease progresses.

❖ **Initial Shock and Grief:** The initial diagnosis often triggers shock and grief for caregivers as they grapple with the reality of their loved one's cognitive decline. The anticipation of changes in the relationship and the uncertainty of the future contribute to a sense of loss.

❖ **Frustration and Helplessness:** As Alzheimer's advances, caregivers may experience frustration and a growing sense of helplessness. Cognitive and behavioral changes in the individual with Alzheimer's can lead to communication challenges, mood swings, and difficulty in managing daily activities, amplifying the caregiver's sense of inadequacy.

❖ **Stress and Burnout:** The demanding nature of caregiving, with constant vigilance, multitasking, and the emotional toll of witnessing a loved one's decline, contributes to chronic stress and burnout. Caregivers may neglect their own needs, leading to physical and emotional exhaustion.

❖ **Guilt and Ambiguous Loss: F**eelings of guilt often arise as caregivers grapple with the inability to provide the level of care they wish to offer. Ambiguous loss, a unique aspect of Alzheimer's caregiving, involves mourning the gradual loss of the person's cognitive and functional abilities while they are physically present.

❖ **Isolation and Loneliness:** The demands of caregiving can lead to social isolation. The stigma surrounding Alzheimer's may contribute to a sense of loneliness, as caregivers may withdraw from social interactions due to difficulties in explaining or managing their loved one's behavior.

❖ **Emotional Resilience and Moments of Joy:** Despite the challenges, caregivers often demonstrate remarkable emotional resilience. Moments of joy and connection, such as shared memories or fleeting instances of recognition, become precious.

These moments provide emotional sustenance amid the difficulties of caregiving.

❖ **Role Reversal and Identity Shift:** Caregivers experience a significant shift in roles as they transition from a traditional relationship dynamic to assuming responsibilities traditionally held by the person with Alzheimer's. This role reversal can evoke complex emotions, challenging the caregiver's sense of identity and purpose.

❖ **Anticipatory Grief:** Anticipatory grief, mourning the loss of the person before their physical death, is a prevalent emotion for caregivers. Witnessing the gradual decline prompts a continuous grieving process as they navigate the changing landscape of their relationship.

❖ **Need for Emotional Support:** The emotional impact underscores the critical need for emotional support for caregivers. Support groups, counseling, and respite care play vital roles in helping caregivers cope with the multifaceted emotional challenges they face. Open communication with healthcare professionals and accessing community resources can alleviate the emotional burden.

Understanding and addressing the emotional impact on caregivers is pivotal for their well-being and the quality of care provided.

Coping strategies for families

Coping with Alzheimer's disease as a family involves navigating various challenges and adapting to the evolving needs of the affected individual. Here are key coping strategies that families can employ;

- ❖ **Education and Information:** Understanding Alzheimer's disease is fundamental. Families benefit from educating themselves about the disease's progression, symptoms, and available resources. Knowledge empowers families to make informed decisions and plan for the future.

- ❖ **Communication:** Open and honest communication within the family is crucial. Discussing expectations, sharing responsibilities, and addressing emotional concerns fosters a supportive environment. Encouraging family members to express their feelings and concerns helps in managing the emotional impact of caregiving.

❖ **Establishing Routines:** Creating consistent routines provides stability for individuals with Alzheimer's. Predictability in daily activities can reduce anxiety and enhance the person's sense of security. Routines also help caregivers plan and organize their tasks effectively.

❖ **Seeking Professional Support:** Engaging with healthcare professionals, including neurologists, geriatricians, and social workers, provides valuable insights and support. Professional guidance aids families in making informed decisions, accessing appropriate care, and navigating the complexities of Alzheimer's.

❖ **Respite Care:** Caregivers often face burnout, emphasizing the importance of respite care. Taking breaks and allowing other family members to share caregiving responsibilities can prevent exhaustion and enhance the overall well-being of caregivers.

❖ **Joining Support Groups:** Support groups offer a platform for families to connect with others facing similar challenges. Sharing experiences, exchanging advice, and learning coping strategies from peers can alleviate feelings of isolation and provide emotional support.

❖ **Legal and Financial Planning:** Addressing legal and financial matters early on is essential. Families should consider establishing power of attorney, discussing long-term care plans, and ensuring financial arrangements are in place. Planning ahead provides a roadmap for managing future challenges.

❖ **Fostering Quality Time:** Despite the challenges, finding moments for quality time with the individual with Alzheimer's is crucial. Engaging in activities that bring joy, reminiscing about shared memories, and fostering connections contribute to a positive and meaningful caregiving experience.

❖ **Self-Care:** Prioritizing self-care is not only important for individual well-being but also benefits the entire family. Caregivers must recognize their own needs, seek support when necessary, and maintain their physical and mental health to sustain the demands of caregiving.

Coping with Alzheimer's as a family involves a collective effort, emphasizing understanding, communication, and a proactive approach to care. By implementing these coping strategies, families can enhance their resilience, support the affected individual, and navigate the journey of Alzheimer's disease with compassion and strength.

Chapter eight

Diet and Lifestyle

Nutrition plays a pivotal role in managing Alzheimer's disease, influencing both cognitive function and overall well-being. A balanced diet rich in antioxidants, omega-3 fatty acids, and vitamins contributes to brain health. Antioxidants, found in fruits and vegetables, combat oxidative stress linked to Alzheimer's pathology. Omega-3 fatty acids, prevalent in fish and nuts, support cognitive function and reduce inflammation. Adequate intake of vitamins, especially B-complex vitamins and vitamin D, is essential for maintaining brain health. Additionally, a diet low in saturated fats and refined sugars helps manage cardiovascular health, reducing the risk of vascular-related cognitive decline. Hydration is equally crucial, as dehydration can exacerbate cognitive symptoms. While nutrition is not a cure, adopting a brain-healthy diet is a proactive measure that supports overall health and may contribute to the management of Alzheimer's disease symptoms.

Nutrition's role in managing Alzheimer's disease

Nutrition plays a crucial role in managing Alzheimer's disease, influencing cognitive function, overall health, and potentially impacting the progression of the condition. A well-balanced diet has the potential to enhance brain health and support individuals affected by Alzheimer's in various ways.

- o **Antioxidant-Rich Foods:** Antioxidants, found in fruits and vegetables, play a vital role in combating oxidative stress associated with Alzheimer's disease. These compounds neutralize free radicals, reducing cellular damage in the brain. Berries, leafy greens, and colorful vegetables are excellent sources of antioxidants.

○ **Omega-3 Fatty Acids:** Omega-3 fatty acids, abundant in fatty fish, flaxseeds, and walnuts, have been associated with cognitive benefits. These essential fatty acids contribute to the structural integrity of brain cell membranes and may have anti-inflammatory effects, potentially slowing cognitive decline in Alzheimer's.

○ **B-Complex Vitamins:** B-complex vitamins, including B6, B12, and folate, are crucial for brain health. They support the production of neurotransmitters and help regulate homocysteine levels. Elevated homocysteine is linked to an increased risk of cognitive decline, and adequate B-vitamin intake may help manage this risk.

○ **Vitamin D:** Vitamin D, often referred to as the "sunshine vitamin," is essential for overall health. Emerging research suggests a potential link between vitamin D deficiency and an increased risk of cognitive decline. Sun exposure, fortified foods, and supplements are sources of vitamin D.

○ **Healthy Fats and Low Sugar:** Prioritizing healthy fats, such as those found in olive oil and avocados, while reducing saturated fats, supports cardiovascular health. Conditions like hypertension and diabetes, which are influenced by diet, are known risk factors for cognitive decline, making heart-healthy nutrition crucial for Alzheimer's management.

- o **Hydration:** Proper hydration is often overlooked but is critical for cognitive function. Dehydration can exacerbate cognitive symptoms, so maintaining an adequate fluid intake is essential.

While nutrition alone cannot cure Alzheimer's, adopting a brain-healthy diet is a proactive approach that supports overall well-being and may influence the management of symptoms.

Chapter Nine

Exercise and cognitive health

Regular exercise is closely linked to cognitive health, playing a significant role in promoting overall brain function and potentially reducing the risk of cognitive decline, including conditions like Alzheimer's disease.

- **Improved Blood Flow and Oxygenation:** Exercise enhances cardiovascular health, improving blood flow and oxygen delivery to the brain. This increased circulation supports the growth of new blood vessels and the maintenance of existing ones, fostering a healthy environment for cognitive function.

- **Neurotransmitter Release:** Physical activity triggers the release of neurotransmitters like dopamine and serotonin, which play crucial roles in mood regulation and cognitive function. These chemicals promote a positive mood and can enhance attention, memory, and learning.

- **Neuroplasticity:** Exercise promotes neuroplasticity, the brain's ability to reorganize itself by forming new neural connections. This adaptability is vital for learning and memory, and exercise has been shown to stimulate the growth of neurons in key regions associated with these cognitive functions.

- **Reduction of Inflammatory Markers:** Chronic inflammation is linked to various neurodegenerative conditions. Regular exercise has anti-inflammatory effects, reducing levels of pro-inflammatory markers. This anti-inflammatory environment may contribute to the preservation of cognitive function.

- **Mitigation of Cardiovascular Risk Factors:** Many risk factors for cardiovascular disease, such as hypertension, diabetes, and high cholesterol, are also risk factors for cognitive decline. Exercise helps manage these cardiovascular risk factors, indirectly supporting cognitive health.

- **Stress Reduction:** Chronic stress can negatively impact cognitive function. Exercise is a natural stress reliever, promoting the release of endorphins, which act as mood elevators. Stress reduction contributes to better cognitive resilience and mental well-being.

- **Cognitive Reserve:** Regular exercise is associated with the development of cognitive reserve. This reserve represents the brain's ability to withstand damage and continue functioning despite age-related changes or disease. Individuals with higher cognitive reserve often exhibit better cognitive performance and resilience.

- **Social Engagement**: Exercise often involves social interaction, whether through group classes, walking with a friend, or participating in team sports. Social engagement is a crucial component of cognitive health, providing mental stimulation and emotional support.

Incorporating regular physical activity into one's routine, such as brisk walking, jogging, swimming, or strength training, can have positive effects on cognitive health.

Chapter Ten

Research and Innovations

Research and innovations in Alzheimer's disease aim to uncover the underlying causes, develop effective treatments, and enhance caregiving approaches. Advances include exploring disease-modifying therapies targeting beta-amyloid and tau proteins, investigating potential biomarkers for early detection, and harnessing technology for monitoring and intervention. Ongoing efforts also focus on understanding genetic influences, exploring lifestyle factors, and improving support systems for individuals and their families. These multifaceted research initiatives offer hope for breakthroughs that may revolutionize our understanding of Alzheimer's and lead to innovative strategies for prevention, early intervention, and improved quality of life for those affected.

Current advancements in Alzheimer's research

Current advancements in Alzheimer's research showcase a dynamic landscape, combining insights from genetics, molecular biology, and innovative technologies to unravel the complexities of the disease. Several key areas are witnessing notable progress:

➢ **Biomarkers and Early Detection:**
Researchers are actively identifying biomarkers that may indicate the early stages of Alzheimer's before symptoms manifest. Advances in imaging techniques, cerebrospinal fluid analysis, and blood-based biomarkers offer promising avenues for early detection, enabling timely interventions.

➢ **Immunotherapy and Targeted Therapies:**
Immunotherapeutic approaches targeting beta-amyloid and tau, the hallmark proteins in Alzheimer's pathology, are undergoing rigorous clinical trials. These treatments aim to modify disease progression by reducing

the accumulation of abnormal protein aggregates in the brain.

➢ **Genetic Insights:** Genetic studies have identified risk factors associated with Alzheimer's, including specific gene variants. Understanding these genetic links provides valuable insights into the disease's mechanisms and informs potential targets for therapeutic interventions.

➢ **Precision Medicine:** The concept of precision medicine tailors treatments based on an individual's unique genetic and molecular profile. This approach holds promise in developing personalized interventions that address the specific characteristics of each person's Alzheimer's disease.

➢ **Artificial Intelligence and Digital Biomarkers**: Innovations in artificial intelligence (AI) are contributing to the analysis of large datasets, aiding in the identification of patterns and trends related to Alzheimer's. Digital biomarkers, including cognitive assessments and wearable technology, provide real-time data for monitoring cognitive changes and disease progression.

➢ **Lifestyle Interventions:** Research explores the impact of lifestyle factors such as diet, exercise, and cognitive stimulation on Alzheimer's risk. Comprehensive interventions focusing on healthy living may offer preventive strategies or contribute to slowing disease progression.

➢ **Global Collaborative Initiatives:** Collaborative efforts on a global scale, like the Alzheimer's Disease Neuroimaging Initiative (ADNI) and the World Wide Alzheimer's Disease Neuroimaging Initiative (WW-ADNI), facilitate data sharing and accelerate the pace of research by pooling resources and expertise.

While breakthroughs in Alzheimer's research are continually emerging, challenges remain. Developing effective disease-modifying therapies, enhancing early detection methods, and addressing the heterogeneity of Alzheimer's presentations are ongoing priorities. Research efforts underscore a commitment to understanding, treating, and ultimately preventing Alzheimer's disease, offering hope for future advancements that may transform the landscape of care and support for affected individuals and their families.

Potential future treatments

Potential future treatments for Alzheimer's disease hold promise for addressing the underlying mechanisms of the condition and revolutionizing therapeutic approaches. Several avenues of research are being explored:

- **Disease-Modifying Therapies:** Advances in understanding the molecular basis of Alzheimer's are paving the way for disease-modifying therapies. Targeting beta-amyloid plaques and tau tangles, the primary pathological hallmarks, remains a focus. Monoclonal antibodies, small molecules, and other approaches aim to reduce or eliminate these protein aggregates to slow or halt disease progression.

- **Neuroprotective Agents:** Researchers are investigating compounds with neuroprotective properties that could shield brain cells from damage. These agents may enhance cellular resilience, improve synaptic function, and mitigate the effects of inflammation associated with Alzheimer's disease.

- **Precision Medicine and Genetic Therapies:** Advances in understanding the genetic factors contributing to Alzheimer's risk open the door to precision medicine approaches. Tailoring treatments based on an individual's genetic profile may lead to more targeted and effective interventions. Genetic therapies, including gene editing techniques, hold potential for modifying disease-related genes.

- **Anti-Inflammatory Drugs:** Chronic inflammation is implicated in Alzheimer's disease progression. Anti-inflammatory drugs, both existing medications and novel compounds, are being explored for their potential to modulate immune responses and reduce neuroinflammation.

- **Mitochondrial Function Modulation:** Dysfunction in mitochondrial function has been observed in Alzheimer's. Future treatments may focus on restoring or enhancing mitochondrial function to support energy production in brain cells, potentially slowing the degenerative processes.

- **Epigenetic Approaches:** Epigenetic modifications influence gene expression without altering the underlying DNA sequence. Emerging research investigates the potential of epigenetic therapies to modify gene activity associated with Alzheimer's, providing a novel avenue for intervention.

- **Cognitive Enhancers and Synaptic Modulators:** Drugs designed to enhance cognitive function and modulate synaptic activity are being explored. These treatments aim to improve memory, attention, and learning abilities, addressing the cognitive deficits characteristic of Alzheimer's.

While these potential future treatments offer hope, it's important to acknowledge the complexity of Alzheimer's disease. The multifaceted nature of the condition requires a comprehensive and nuanced approach. Clinical trials and ongoing research will continue to refine these potential treatments, with the ultimate goal of providing more effective and targeted interventions to address the diverse aspects of Alzheimer's and enhance the quality of life for those affected.

Chapter Eleven

Support Systems

Support systems for individuals with Alzheimer's encompass a network of care, resources, and understanding. This includes family, friends, and caregivers who provide emotional and practical assistance. Support groups offer a space for shared experiences and advice. Healthcare professionals, including neurologists and social workers, contribute expertise. Community programs and organizations provide educational resources and services. Robust support systems enhance the well-being of both individuals with Alzheimer's and their caregivers, fostering a collaborative environment to navigate the challenges associated with the disease.

Community resources

Community resources play a vital role in supporting individuals affected by Alzheimer's disease and their caregivers. These resources are designed to provide assistance, education, and a sense of community, contributing to the overall well-being of those navigating the challenges of Alzheimer's.

> **Alzheimer's Associations and Helplines:** Local and national Alzheimer's associations offer a wealth of information, support groups, and helplines. These organizations provide a valuable connection for individuals seeking guidance, resources, and a sense of community.

> **Memory Cafés and Social Programs:** Memory cafés and social programs create inclusive spaces where individuals with Alzheimer's and their caregivers can engage in activities, share experiences, and build connections. These initiatives foster a supportive environment and reduce social isolation.

➢ **Respite Care Services:** Respite care services provide temporary relief for caregivers, offering professional care for individuals with Alzheimer's. This allows caregivers the opportunity to rest, attend to personal needs, and reduce the risk of burnout.

➢ **Educational Workshops and Training:** Community organizations often host educational workshops and training sessions for caregivers. These programs cover a range of topics, including understanding Alzheimer's, effective communication strategies, and practical caregiving techniques.

➢ **Transportation Services:** Transportation services catered to individuals with Alzheimer's ensure safe and reliable travel to medical appointments, community events, and social gatherings. These services contribute to maintaining a sense of independence and engagement in the community.

➢ **Adult Day Programs:** Adult day programs offer structured activities and supervision for individuals with Alzheimer's. These programs provide cognitive stimulation, social interaction, and respite for caregivers, promoting overall well-being.

> **Legal and Financial Assistance:** Community resources often include services that offer legal and financial guidance. Assistance with legal matters, financial planning, and accessing benefits helps families navigate the complexities associated with Alzheimer's care.

> **Supportive Housing and Care Facilities:** Supportive housing options and care facilities tailored to individuals with Alzheimer's provide a secure and supportive environment. These facilities often offer specialized care and programs designed to meet the unique needs of individuals with memory impairment.

Community resources serve as crucial pillars of support for individuals affected by Alzheimer's and their families. By offering a range of services, these resources contribute to a more informed, connected, and resilient community, empowering individuals to navigate the complexities of Alzheimer's disease with dignity and support.

The role of support organizations and groups

Support groups and organizations dedicated to Alzheimer's disease provide invaluable resources, community, and assistance for individuals facing the challenges of this neurodegenerative condition. These groups play a crucial role in fostering emotional well-being, sharing knowledge, and offering practical support for both individuals with Alzheimer's and their caregivers.

1. **Emotional Support:** Alzheimer's support groups create a safe space for individuals to express their emotions, fears, and challenges openly. Connecting with others facing similar experiences helps reduce feelings of isolation and provides emotional support.

2. **Information and Education:** Organizations focused on Alzheimer's offer comprehensive information and educational resources. This includes materials on understanding the disease, available treatments, caregiving strategies,

and coping mechanisms. Access to reliable information empowers individuals and caregivers to make informed decisions.

3. **Caregiver Guidance:** Support groups often include specialized sessions for caregivers, addressing the unique challenges they face. Caregiver support provides a platform to share practical tips, discuss caregiving strategies, and offer guidance on managing the complex aspects of daily life.

4. **Advocacy and Awareness:** Alzheimer's organizations actively engage in advocacy efforts to raise awareness, influence public policy, and advance research initiatives. By amplifying the voices of those affected, these groups contribute to shaping a more supportive and informed society.

5. **Practical Resources:** Support organizations offer practical resources such as toolkits, guides, and checklists for managing various aspects of Alzheimer's care. These resources cover legal and financial considerations, safety measures, and tips for enhancing the quality of life for individuals with Alzheimer's.

6. **Helplines and Crisis Intervention:** Many organizations operate helplines and crisis intervention services, providing immediate assistance and guidance during challenging situations. These services offer a lifeline for individuals and caregivers facing urgent concerns.

7. **Research and Clinical Trials:** Alzheimer's support organizations often collaborate with researchers and facilitate participation in clinical trials. By connecting individuals with research opportunities, these groups contribute to the advancement of treatments and potential cures.

8. **Community Engagement:** Local support groups organize community events, memory walks, and educational sessions. These activities foster a sense of community, allowing individuals and caregivers to connect, share experiences, and build a support network within their local area.

Support groups and organizations create a collaborative and understanding network for those affected by Alzheimer's. By addressing the emotional, informational, and practical needs of individuals and caregivers, these groups play a pivotal role in enhancing the quality of life and promoting resilience in the face of Alzheimer's disease.

Chapter Twelve

Legal and Financial Planning

Legal and financial planning is crucial for individuals and families navigating Alzheimer's disease. Establishing power of attorney, advance directives, and wills ensures decision-making continuity. Financial planning involves organizing assets, exploring insurance options, and preparing for long-term care costs. Engaging legal and financial professionals early on provides a roadmap for managing complexities, protecting assets, and addressing potential challenges associated with Alzheimer's care, offering peace of mind for individuals and their families.

Legal considerations for families

Legal considerations for families dealing with Alzheimer's disease involve essential planning to address various aspects of care and decision making. Here are key considerations

1. **Power of Attorney (POA):** Establishing a durable power of attorney allows individuals to designate a trusted person to make financial and legal decisions on their behalf if they become incapacitated. This ensures a seamless transition of decision-making authority.

2. **Advance Directives:** Advance directives, including living wills and healthcare proxies, articulate an individual's preferences regarding medical treatment and end-of-life care. This legal documentation guides healthcare decisions when the person with Alzheimer's may no longer communicate their wishes.

3. **Guardianship:** In situations where an individual with Alzheimer's has not designated a power of attorney, and cognitive impairment prevents effective decision-making, guardianship may be considered. This involves a legal process where a court appoints a guardian to make decisions on behalf of the person with Alzheimer's.

4. **Estate Planning**: Comprehensive estate planning includes creating or updating wills, trusts, and other legal documents to ensure the orderly distribution of assets. This process can also help minimize tax implications and provide financial security for family members.

5. **Long-Term Care Planning:** Legal considerations for long-term care involve exploring options such as Medicaid planning, securing long-term care insurance, and understanding the legal implications of various care settings. Planning for long-term care can help families navigate the financial challenges associated with Alzheimer's care.

6. **Financial Management:** Families should establish a clear financial management plan, including budgeting for current and anticipated expenses related to Alzheimer's care. This may involve working with financial advisors to ensure proper asset management and protection.

7. **Legal Consultation:** Seeking legal advice early in the Alzheimer's journey is crucial. A

legal professional with expertise in elder law and estate planning can provide tailored guidance based on the family's unique circumstances, ensuring that legal arrangements align with the specific needs of the individual with Alzheimer's and their family.

8. **Family Communication:** Open and transparent communication within the family is essential. Discussing legal considerations and plans ensures that everyone is on the same page and understands the decisions made regarding the care and future of the individual with Alzheimer's.

Navigating the legal aspects of Alzheimer's care demands thoughtful planning and consultation with legal professionals. By addressing these considerations proactively, families can establish a solid foundation that supports the well-being of the individual with Alzheimer's and provides clarity and support for family members involved in the caregiving journey.

Financial planning for long-term care

Financial planning for long-term care is a critical aspect for families dealing with Alzheimer's disease, considering the potential high costs associated with specialized care. Here are key considerations:

✓ **Assessing Current Finances:** Begin by evaluating the individual's current financial situation, including income, savings, investments, and insurance coverage. This assessment provides a foundation for understanding available resources.

✓ **Long-Term Care Insurance:** Explore long-term care insurance options early. Policies vary, covering expenses such as in-home care, assisted living, or nursing home care. Purchasing insurance before the onset of cognitive decline is advisable, as coverage may be limited or more costly with a pre-existing condition.

✓ **Medicaid Planning:** Medicaid can help cover long-term care costs, but eligibility requirements and regulations vary by state. Engage in Medicaid planning early to understand requirements and navigate the application process.

✓ **Estate Planning and Asset Protection:** Estate planning, including creating trusts and updating wills, can help protect assets and streamline their distribution. Certain legal tools may also be utilized to safeguard assets from the high costs of long-term care.

✓ **Budgeting for Care:** Develop a comprehensive budget that accounts for current and anticipated long-term care expenses. Consider potential costs for home modifications, medical equipment, and professional caregiving services.

✓ **Utilizing Veterans Benefits:** Veterans and their spouses may qualify for benefits, including Aid and Attendance, which can help offset long-term care costs. Understanding available veterans' benefits is crucial for maximizing financial support.

✓ **Family Contributions and Support:** Discuss financial contributions from family members willing and able to contribute to the cost of care. Open communication can help distribute responsibilities and alleviate the financial burden on a single individual.

✓ **Professional Financial Advice:** Consult with financial advisors who specialize in elder care and long-term planning. Professionals can provide guidance on investment strategies, tax implications, and optimizing available resources to meet the evolving needs of Alzheimer's care.

✓ **Consideration of Public Programs:** Investigate public programs and community resources that may offer financial assistance for specific aspects of long-term care. These may include home and community-based services that can support individuals with Alzheimer's in their preferred living environment.

Navigating the financial aspects of long-term care for Alzheimer's requires careful planning and a proactive approach. Families should seek professional advice, explore available resources, and develop a comprehensive financial strategy that aligns with the specific needs and preferences of the individual with Alzheimer's. Planning early allows families to make informed decisions and create a financial safety net for the challenges that may arise in the course of Alzheimer's care.

Chapter Thirteen

Quality of Life

Quality of life for individuals affected by Alzheimer's extends beyond medical care to encompass emotional well-being, independence, and meaningful connections. Maintaining a high quality of life involves personalized care, social engagement, and support systems tailored to the individual's preferences. Meaningful activities, compassionate relationships, and a supportive environment contribute to a sense of purpose, fostering a dignified and fulfilling life despite the challenges posed by Alzheimer's. Prioritizing quality of life underscores the importance of holistic care that addresses not only the physical aspects of the disease but also the emotional and social dimensions, enriching the overall well-being of those affected.

Enhancing well-being for individuals with Alzheimer's involves a holistic approach that prioritizes physical, emotional, and social dimensions of care.

1. **Person-Centered Care:** Tailoring care to individual preferences and needs is fundamental. Understanding the person's history, interests, and values allows for personalized engagement, contributing to a sense of identity and well-being.

2. **Meaningful Activities:** Incorporating meaningful activities fosters a sense of purpose. Activities aligned with past interests or current capabilities, such as music, art, or reminiscence therapy, provide cognitive stimulation and emotional fulfillment.

3. **Social Engagement:** Maintaining social connections is crucial. Regular interaction with family, friends, and caregivers helps prevent isolation. Group activities and support networks create a sense of belonging, reducing feelings of loneliness.

4. **Physical Exercise:** Regular physical activity has cognitive and emotional benefits. Adapted exercises, such as walking or chair

yoga, support mobility, enhance mood, and contribute to overall well-being.

5. **Nutritional Support:** Proper nutrition is vital for physical health and cognitive function. Well-balanced, nutrient-rich meals support overall well-being. Addressing dietary preferences and ensuring hydration are essential components of care.

6. **Sensory Stimulation:** Engaging multiple senses through sensory stimulation can enhance cognitive function and emotional well-being. This includes activities like aromatherapy, tactile experiences, and exposure to nature.

7. **Calming Environments:** Creating calming and familiar environments reduces stress and anxiety. Limiting noise, using soft lighting, and incorporating familiar objects contribute to a sense of security and comfort.

8. **Dignified Communication:** Respectful and dignified communication is paramount. Using clear and simple language, maintaining eye contact, and allowing time

for responses fosters positive interactions and preserves the individual's dignity.

In summary, enhancing well-being for individuals with Alzheimer's involves a comprehensive and individualized approach. By prioritizing person-centered care, meaningful activities, social connections, and physical health, caregivers contribute to a higher quality of life, promoting dignity and enriching the overall experience for those navigating Alzheimer's disease.

Creative therapies and activities

Creative therapies and activities play a significant role in enhancing the well-being of individuals with Alzheimer's, offering avenues for self-expression, cognitive stimulation, and emotional engagement.

- ✓ **Art Therapy:** Art therapy provides a non-verbal means of expression. Individuals can engage in painting, drawing, or other artistic activities, fostering creativity and allowing them to communicate emotions and memories.

✓ **Music Therapy:** Music has a profound impact on individuals with Alzheimer's. Music therapy involves listening to familiar tunes, singing, or playing instruments. It can evoke memories, reduce anxiety, and enhance mood, contributing to emotional well-being.

✓ **Reminiscence Therapy:** Encouraging individuals to recall and share past experiences through reminiscence therapy fosters a sense of identity and connection. This can be facilitated through photo albums, storytelling, or memory-sharing sessions.

✓ **Dance and Movement:** Dance and movement therapies offer both physical exercise and emotional expression. Adapted dance routines or simple movements to music can enhance mobility, balance, and emotional well-being.

✓ **Horticulture Therapy:** Engaging individuals in gardening or nature-related activities provides a sensory-rich experience. Planting, tending to flowers, or enjoying outdoor spaces can promote relaxation and connection with the natural world.

✓ **Pet Therapy:** Interactions with animals, known as pet therapy, have shown positive effects on individuals with Alzheimer's. Whether through visits from therapy animals or having a pet, this can alleviate stress, enhance mood, and provide companionship.

✓ **Storytelling and Drama:** Storytelling and drama activities allow individuals to engage in creative expression. This may involve acting out stories, participating in group storytelling, or engaging in simple dramatic exercises to stimulate imagination.

✓ **Multi-Sensory Experiences:** Creating multi-sensory experiences involves stimulating various senses simultaneously. This can include scented oils, textured objects, and soothing sounds, providing a rich and engaging environment.

✓ **Poetry and Writing:** Engaging in poetry or writing activities provides an outlet for self-expression. Whether through journaling, writing short stories, or participating in poetry sessions, individuals can communicate thoughts and emotions.

✓ **Culinary Activities:** Simple culinary activities, such as baking or cooking, offer sensory stimulation and a sense of accomplishment. In addition to the joy of creating something, individuals may find comfort and connection through familiar tastes and smells.

These creative therapies and activities contribute to the overall well-being of individuals with Alzheimer's by promoting engagement, self-expression, and connection.

Chapter Fourteen

Global perspective

Global perspectives on Alzheimer's underscore the need for collaborative efforts in research, care, and advocacy. Recognizing the universal impact of the disease, countries worldwide are working together to share knowledge, promote awareness, and advance research initiatives. Cross-cultural understanding informs diverse caregiving approaches, considering varied societal norms and support structures. Global perspectives emphasize the importance of equitable access to resources, fostering a collective commitment to enhancing the quality of life for individuals affected by Alzheimer's on an international scale.

Alzheimer's impact on a global scale

Alzheimer's disease exerts a profound impact on a global scale, presenting significant challenges to healthcare systems, economies, and societies worldwide. As populations age, the prevalence of Alzheimer's continues to rise, contributing to a growing global health crisis.

1. **Economic Burden:** Alzheimer's imposes a substantial economic burden on nations. Costs associated with healthcare, long-term care, and lost productivity due to caregiving demands are staggering. The financial strain extends to families, affecting their ability to provide adequate care and support.

2. **Healthcare Systems:** The increasing prevalence of Alzheimer's places strain on healthcare systems globally. Diagnosis, treatment, and long-term care demand substantial resources, highlighting the importance of robust healthcare infrastructure to address the complex needs of affected individuals.

3. **Caregiver Impact:** Alzheimer's profoundly affects family members and caregivers. The

emotional, physical, and financial toll on those providing care is substantial. The global caregiving community faces common challenges related to stigma, limited support systems, and the need for accessible resources.

4. **Societal Challenges:** Alzheimer's contributes to broader societal challenges, including changing family dynamics, workforce productivity losses, and strained social support networks. As the disease progresses, individuals may require increasing levels of care, impacting the overall fabric of communities.

In summary, Alzheimer's disease transcends geographical boundaries, affecting individuals, families, and societies worldwide. Recognizing the global impact underscores the importance of collaborative efforts in research, caregiving, and policy development to address the challenges posed by this prevalent and complex neurodegenerative condition.

Chapter Fifteen

Glossary

Alzheimer's Disease: A progressive neurodegenerative disorder characterized by cognitive decline, memory loss, and impaired daily functioning. It is the most common cause of dementia.

Dementia: A broad term encompassing various cognitive impairments affecting memory, reasoning, and daily activities. Alzheimer's is a common cause of dementia.

Neurodegeneration: The progressive loss of structure or function of neurons, leading to cognitive decline and other neurological symptoms seen in Alzheimer's disease.

Beta-Amyloid: Abnormal protein fragments that accumulate in the brains of individuals with

Alzheimer's, forming plaques that contribute to neuronal damage.

Tau Proteins: Proteins involved in maintaining the structure of brain cells. In Alzheimer's, abnormal tau proteins accumulate and form tangles, disrupting cell function.

Cognition: Mental processes related to acquiring knowledge, including memory, attention, language, problem-solving, and perception.

Hippocampus: A brain region crucial for memory formation and consolidation. It is particularly affected in the early stages of Alzheimer's disease.

Neurons: Nerve cells responsible for transmitting information within the brain and nervous system.

Amyloid Plaques: Clumps of beta-amyloid proteins that accumulate between nerve cells in the brain, disrupting communication and contributing to Alzheimer's pathology.

Neurofibrillary Tangles: Twisted, abnormal clumps of tau proteins found within brain cells, a hallmark of Alzheimer's disease.

Mild Cognitive Impairment (MCI): A stage between normal age-related cognitive decline and ore severe cognitive impairment. Some individuals with MCI progress to Alzheimer's disease.

Early-Onset Alzheimer's: Alzheimer's disease diagnosed before the age of 65. It is relatively rare and often has a stronger genetic component.

Late-Onset Alzheimer's: The more common form of Alzheimer's diagnosed after the age of 65, with no clear genetic cause.

Vascular Dementia: Dementia caused by impaired blood flow to the brain, often due to strokes or other vascular issues.

Lewy Body Dementia: A type of dementia characterized by abnormal protein deposits called Lewy bodies, leading to cognitive and motor symptoms.

Frontotemporal Dementia: Dementia that primarily affects the frontal and temporal lobes of the brain, leading to changes in personality, behavior, and language.

Geriatrician: Healthcare professional specializing in the care of older adults, including the diagnosis and management of conditions like Alzheimer's.

Palliative Care: Specialized medical care focused on providing relief from symptoms and improving the quality of life for individuals with serious illnesses, including Alzheimer's.

Respite Care: Short-term care provided to individuals with Alzheimer's, giving their primary caregivers a temporary break.

Caregiver Burnout: Physical, emotional, and mental exhaustion experienced by individuals providing extensive care to someone with Alzheimer's.

Sundowning: Behavioral changes and increased confusion that often occur in the late afternoon or evening in individuals with Alzheimer's.

Advance Directives: Legal documents outlining an individual's preferences for medical treatment in case they become unable to communicate their wishes.

Power of Attorney: Legal authorization for someone to make decisions on behalf of another person, often used in healthcare and financial matters for individuals with Alzheimer's.

Memory Care: Specialized care services designed to meet the unique needs of individuals with Alzheimer's and other forms of dementia.

Assisted Living: Residential facilities providing support for daily living activities, suitable for individuals in the early stages of Alzheimer's.

Long-Term Care Insurance: - Insurance policies covering the costs of long-term care services, including those required for individuals with Alzheimer's.

Clinical Trials: Research studies involving human participants to evaluate new treatments or interventions for Alzheimer's disease.

Neurologist: A medical doctor specializing in the diagnosis and treatment of disorders affecting the nervous system, including Alzheimer's.

Cognitive Reserve: - The brain's ability to withstand damage and function despite the presence of pathology. Activities like education and intellectual stimulation contribute to szcognitive reserve.

Rehabilitation Therapies: Therapeutic interventions, such as physical, occupational, or speech therapy, aimed at improving or maintaining functioning in individuals with Alzheimer's.

Gerontologist: A professional specializing in the study of aging, providing expertise in the physical, mental, and social aspects of aging.

Genomic Studies: Research exploring the role of genetics in Alzheimer's disease to identify risk factors and potential genetic contributors.

Global Initiative on Alzheimer's Disease (GIA): - Collaborative efforts, often led by international organizations, aimed at addressing Alzheimer's challenges on a global scale.

Behavioral Interventions: Approaches targeting behavioral symptoms of Alzheimer's, including agitation and aggression, through non-pharmacological means.

Functional MRI (fMRI): Brain imaging technique measuring changes in blood flow to identify brain regions associated with specific cognitive functions.

Geriatric Psychiatry: Psychiatry specializing in the mental health and emotional well-being of older adults, often addressing conditions like Alzheimer's.

Anticholinesterase Inhibitors: Medications used to temporarily improve cognitive symptoms in Alzheimer's by increasing the levels of acetylcholine, a neurotransmitter.

NMDA Receptor Antagonists: Medications that regulate glutamate levels in the brain, used in Alzheimer's to manage cognitive symptoms.

Non-Pharmacological Therapies: - Therapeutic interventions that do not involve medications, such as music therapy, art therapy, and behavioral interventions.

Geriatric Assessment: Comprehensive evaluation of an older individual's physical health, mental health, and functional status, often performed by a geriatrician.

Conclusion

In traversing the intricate landscape of Alzheimer's disease, we have explored the myriad facets that shape its impact on individuals, families, and societies. As we conclude this journey, it is essential to recap key points and illuminate the pathways of hope that inspire our collective dedication to a future where Alzheimer's is understood, managed, and ultimately conquered.

Recap of Key Points

Our exploration began with an overview of Alzheimer's disease, unraveling its historical context, discoveries, and the intricate web of its impact on global health. We delved into the molecular intricacies of beta-amyloid and tau proteins, the neurodegenerative culprits that weave the complex narrative of cognitive decline. Through the stages of Alzheimer's, we witnessed the progression of symptoms, from early signs and symptoms to the intricate tapestry of the disease's pathology.

Understanding the diverse types of Alzheimer's, including early-onset and familial forms, highlighted the need for personalized approaches to care and research. The global perspective underscored the universality of Alzheimer's impact, necessitating collaborative efforts, research networks, and shared knowledge to address the challenges it poses to healthcare systems and societies worldwide.

We explored the importance of early detection, diagnostic tools, and the pivotal role they play in shaping interventions. The journey unfolded into the nuanced realms of caregiving, emotional impacts on caregivers, and strategies to cope with the challenges posed by Alzheimer's. We examined the significance of nutrition, exercise, and holistic care approaches that enrich the quality of life for individuals navigating the complexities of Alzheimer's.

Financial planning, legal considerations, and the imperative role of support systems became focal points, recognizing the importance of comprehensive strategies in managing the multifaceted dimensions of Alzheimer's. The glossary provided a navigational guide through the terminological landscape, ensuring clarity and understanding for readers engaging with the complexities of Alzheimer's disease.

Hope for the Future

Amid the challenges that Alzheimer's presents, there is a beacon of hope illuminating the path forward. Research initiatives, propelled by international collaborations, continue to deepen our understanding of Alzheimer's. From genomic studies to clinical trials, the scientific community is forging new avenues that hold promise for innovative treatments and interventions.

The evolving landscape of Alzheimer's care witnesses the emergence of holistic approaches, including non-pharmacological interventions, creative therapies, and personalized care plans. These strategies emphasize the importance of preserving dignity, enhancing well-being, and fostering meaningful connections for individuals affected by Alzheimer's.

Advancements in technology, neuroimaging, and biomarker research offer glimpses into the early stages of Alzheimer's, opening windows for timely interventions and preventive measures. The field of precision medicine holds potential to tailor treatments based on individual genetic profiles, paving the way for more effective and personalized care.

As we stand at the intersection of the present and the future, it is crucial to recognize the resilience of individuals, families, and communities affected by Alzheimer's. The power of advocacy movements, increased public awareness, and the commitment of healthcare professionals create a foundation upon which we can build a more compassionate and informed society.